Schizop

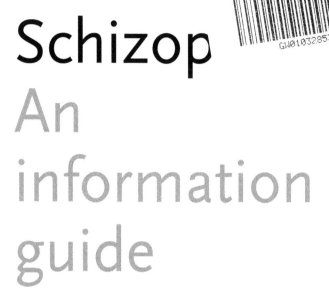

An
information
guide

Debbie Ernest, MSW, RSW
Olga Vuksic, RN, MScN
Ashley Shepard-Smith, MSW, RSW
Emily Webb, MScOT, OT Reg. (Ont.)

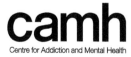

camh
Centre for Addiction and Mental Health

A Pan American Health Organization /
World Health Organization Collaborating Centre

Library and Archives Canada Cataloguing in Publication

Ernest, Debbie, 1970-, author
    Schizophrenia : an information guide / Debbie Ernest, MSW, RSW, Olga
Vuksic, RN, MScN, Ashley Shepard-Smith, MSW, RSW, Emily Webb, MScOT, OT
Reg. (Ont.).

Includes bibliographical references.
Issued in print and electronic formats.
ISBN 978-1-77052-619-8 (PAPERBACK).--ISBN 978-1-77052-620-4 (PDF).--ISBN
978-1-77052-621-1 (HTML).--ISBN 978-1-77052-622-8 (EPUB).--ISBN 978-1-77114-
235-9 (KINDLE)

    1. Schizophrenia. I. Vuksic, Olga, 1970-, author II. Shepard-Smith, Ashley,
1986-, author III. Webb, Emily, 1985- author IV. Centre for Addiction and Mental
Health, issuing body V. Title.

RC514.E76 2017   616.89'8   C2017-904354-4
C2017-904355-2

Printed in Canada

This publication may be available in other formats. For information about alternative
formats or other CAMH publications, or to place an order, please contact CAMH
Publications:
Toll-free: 1 800 661-1111
Toronto: 416 595-6059
E-mail: publications@camh.ca
Online store: http://store.camh.ca
Website: www.camh.ca

Disponible en français sous le titre :
La schizophrénie : Guide d'information

This guide was produced by CAMH Education.

3973k / 03-2018 / PM117

Contents

Acknowledgments

The authors thank the people who shared their personal experiences of schizophrenia with us and permitted us to include them in this guide: Ann, Gilda, Moustafa Ragheb, Moshe Sakal and S. We also thank those who reviewed earlier drafts of the guide: patient and family reviewers Ann, Gilda, Moustafa Ragheb, Moshe Sakal, V.C.C. and Henry Yip; and professional reviewers April Collins, MSW, RSW; Sean A. Kidd, PhD, CPsych, CPRP; Yarissa Herman, DPsych, CPsych; Mike Pett, MSW, RSW; Gary Remington, MD, PhD, FRCPC and John Spavor, MSc (OT).

We thank the authors of previous CAMH publications, including other guides in this series, whose work provided a foundation for the information presented here. Thanks in particular to Jane Patterson, Dale Butterill, Claudia Tindall, David Clodman and April Collins, who wrote the earlier edition of this guide.

Thanks finally to the CAMH Education team: Michelle Maynes, product developer; Nick Gamble, editor; and Mara Korkola, designer.

Introduction

This guide is for people with schizophrenia, their families and friends, and anyone else interested in better understanding the illness and what it is like to experience it.

The guide should answer many of the questions you may have about schizophrenia. It can also help you to know what questions to ask treatment providers. You may wish to read it from beginning to end, or to dip into it. Keep in mind, though, that some terms and concepts are explained in the opening chapters.

We want the guide to promote hope, and to provide information that empowers people with schizophrenia, and their families, to take charge of their treatment and their lives. However, the guide also acknowledges the challenges that schizophrenia can bring. The experience of the illness varies widely depending on the person, the support available to them, and where they are in their recovery journey. The quotations we include from people with experience of schizophrenia illustrate this range of experience.

1 What is schizophrenia?

Some people say that schizophrenia is when people hear voices and see things that aren't there, but for me it was different: I experienced difficult and disturbing thoughts. My thoughts made me do things or say things that are not acceptable. At first it seemed like nothing, but then I wasn't doing well in school, and it became distressing. When I went to university I started thinking people were out to get me. I wasn't able to function; I wasn't able to carry out normal everyday activities. — Ann

Schizophrenia is a complex mental illness that affects how a person thinks, feels, behaves and relates to others. The illness occurs in both men and women, but is slightly more common in men. The first episode typically occurs in the late teens to early twenties—usually earlier for men than for women. People can also develop the illness later in life. As many as one person out of 100 may experience schizophrenia. At any one time, as many as 51 million people worldwide experience schizophrenia, including more than 280,000 people in Canada.

Schizophrenia can be a challenging illness to live with and to understand. Symptoms such as hallucinations and delusions can cause people to lose contact with reality. This experience can be confusing and distressing for the person with schizophrenia, and for family members, friends and others, who often don't understand what is happening or know how to relate to the person who is ill. People with schizophrenia may also experience changes to the way they think and have trouble expressing themselves and managing basic daily tasks. They may become withdrawn and isolated.

Recovery from schizophrenia is a gradual process that is unique to each person. The symptoms usually improve and become easier to manage over time, though they do not always disappear. A recovery-oriented approach to the treatment of schizophrenia promotes the values of hope, empowerment and optimism. The illness can usually be managed effectively with a combination of medications and psychosocial supports, such as psychotherapy, education and peer support. People with schizophrenia can and do recover, and lead meaningful and fulfilling lives.

> *I want others to understand that it is only the worst cases that you see in the news. There are a lot of people who live with it and you wouldn't have any idea they even have it. We are people too. We have feelings. We have endless possibilities, just like anyone.* — S

How does schizophrenia begin and what is its course?

Schizophrenia often starts so gradually that people experiencing symptoms and their families may not be aware of the illness for a long time. For some, however, the symptoms come on rapidly and are more easily recognized. Schizophrenia has three phases: prodromal (or beginning), active and residual. These phases tend to occur in sequence and to repeat in cycles throughout the illness. The length of each phase varies from person to person.

1. PRODROMAL PHASE

When symptoms develop gradually, people may begin to lose interest in their regular activities and withdraw from friends and family members. They may become confused, have trouble concentrating and feel listless and apathetic, preferring to spend most of their days alone. They may also become intensely preoccupied with certain topics or ideas (e.g., persecution, religion, public figures). Family and friends may be upset with this behaviour, not understanding that it is caused by illness. Occasionally, these symptoms reach a plateau and do not develop further but, in most cases, an active phase of the illness follows. The prodromal period can last weeks, months or even years.

2. ACTIVE PHASE

During the active, or acute, phase of the illness, people typically experience symptoms of psychosis, such as delusions, hallucinations, jumbled thoughts, and disturbances in behaviour and feelings. However, these symptoms can also be caused by other mental and physical health conditions (e.g., bipolar disorder, drug-induced psychosis, head injury), and so other factors are considered in diagnosing schizophrenia (see page 10).

The active phase of schizophrenia most often appears after a prodromal period, but sometimes the symptoms can appear suddenly.

3. RESIDUAL PHASE

After an active phase, when symptoms have settled down, people may be listless and withdrawn, and have trouble concentrating. The symptoms in this phase are similar to those in the prodromal phase.

People with schizophrenia may become actively ill just once or twice in their life, or may have many episodes. Unfortunately, after each active phase, residual symptoms may increase and a person's ability to function normally may decrease. This is one reason it is important to try to avoid relapses (the return of active symptoms) by participating in the recommended treatment and recovery plan.

> *You are a totally different person from what people know you as. You just behave completely different. They see you and think: this is not the person I know. Why is he acting like this? But it's from the illness.* —
> Moustafa

What are the symptoms of schizophrenia?

People with schizophrenia experience delusions; hallucinations; disorganized thought, speech or behaviour; and other symptoms that affect their ability to function in their daily activities. Remember though that these symptoms are not specific to schizophrenia— they can also be signs of other mental and physical illnesses.

The main symptoms of schizophrenia are divided into "positive," "negative" and cognitive categories. People with schizophrenia often also experience some other symptoms.

POSITIVE SYMPTOMS

The term "positive" is used to describe symptoms that are "added on" by the illness. Positive symptoms include delusions, hallucinations and disorganized thought, speech and behaviour.

Delusions

Delusions are firmly held false beliefs that have no basis in fact or in the person's culture. The person feels so strongly about these beliefs that they will not accept other people's attempts to argue against or disprove the beliefs. Delusions are sometimes understood to be extreme distortions and/or misinterpretations of the person's perceptions or experiences. Common delusions among people with schizophrenia include the beliefs that:

· other people are following or monitoring them or trying to harm them (also referred to as paranoia)
· their bodies or thoughts are being controlled by outside forces
· ordinary events have special meaning for them (e.g., believing that a newspaper story, song lyric or TV character is communicating special messages intended for them)
· they are especially important or have unusual powers
· other people can read their thoughts.

Hallucinations

Hallucinations are disturbances in perception. If a person hears, sees, tastes, smells or feels something that does not actually exist, they are hallucinating. The most common hallucinations among people with schizophrenia are auditory; that is, they hear noises or voices, often talking to them or about them. These voices may be experienced as harmless, with the voices commenting on things or people around the person. For some, the voices may even be comforting. However, it is more common for the voices to be frightening or humiliating, causing the person to be distressed. Voices may also be experienced as commands—ordering the person to perform some kind of action. How distressing the voices are can depend on what the voices are saying and on the meaning the person makes of what they are hearing.

Disorganized thought and speech

Schizophrenia can affect a person's ability to connect thoughts and to communicate with others in a way that is clear and logical. Their thoughts may be jumbled or blocked, and this is expressed through their speech. For example, when talking, they may:

· jump from subject to subject
· make up words that don't make sense
· talk about ideas that seem to be unrelated
· answer questions in ways that are off-topic or irrelevant
· string together rhyming words that make no sense.

Disorganized behaviour

Schizophrenia can affect a person's ability to complete everyday tasks such as bathing, local travel, basic school and work activities, buying groceries and preparing food. People with schizophrenia may be unable to plan their days and to follow through with ordinary tasks.

They may also behave in ways that seem unusual to others. For example, they may become agitated for no apparent reason, or be uninhibited in social situations.

Less commonly, a person may have "catatonic" symptoms. These may include rigid body posture, motionlessness, excessive repetitive movements or not reacting to their environment.

> For me, schizophrenia is jumbled thoughts and doing things I would not normally do. The last time I was admitted to the hospital, I had thrown my furniture out of my apartment: my bed, my tables, my TV, my radio, my computer, and then my clothes. I called the police every day because things were not going right. My furniture was missing—I was putting out my furniture, but why was I doing that? — Ann

NEGATIVE SYMPTOMS

Negative symptoms of schizophrenia "take away" from a person's usual ability to accomplish tasks and enjoy life. They include reduced motivation, social withdrawal, reduced emotional expression, loss of interest and pleasure, and reduced verbal communication.

Negative symptoms tend to last longer than positive symptoms, and often disrupt the person's ability to work, go to school, take care of others and accomplish daily tasks.

Reduced motivation

A person with schizophrenia may have problems finishing tasks or making and carrying out plans. They may also have less energy and drive, both before and after an active phase of the illness. Some people misinterpret this behaviour as laziness or as "not wanting to try." They may believe the behaviour is intentional, and become frustrated with the person. But this behaviour is related to the illness and not to the person's character.

Social withdrawal

One of the earliest symptoms that many people with schizophrenia experience is a change in their sensitivity toward others. A person may become more sensitive to and aware of other people, or they may withdraw and pay little or no attention to others. The person may become suspicious and worried that others are avoiding them, talking about them or feeling negatively toward them. The person may feel safer and calmer being alone. They may also become so absorbed in their own thoughts and sensations that they lose interest in the feelings and lives of others. They may spend more time alone in their room, not engaging with family or friends.

> *All that happened was that she said: I'm not going to school any more. She couldn't cope with it. She couldn't articulate what she was feeling because she didn't know. I would say, are you okay? And she'd say, yeah. I did not see how much she was struggling. She isolated herself. She was trying to figure it out. She was just in her room. For her it was very inward.* — Gilda

Reduced emotional expression

Many people with schizophrenia tend to have reduced emotional expressiveness. This may be seen in a lack of facial expression, a monotonous voice, fixed or prolonged staring, and less expressive body language than before the illness began.

Loss of interest and pleasure

Interest in things that once brought satisfaction, pleasure or joy is often reduced or lost for people with schizophrenia. This might include activities like playing an instrument, playing a sport or enjoying a hobby, either with others or alone. However, as people start feeling better, these interests may return.

Reduced verbal communication

Slowed or blocked thoughts may cause a person with schizophrenia to speak very little, even in situations where they are expected to speak. Questions may be answered in short phrases with limited content.

Change in habits and ability to function

A person with schizophrenia may lose interest in their appearance, in the way they dress and in grooming and bathing. They may find it difficult to carry out daily activities such as shopping or going to work.

COGNITIVE AND OTHER SYMPTOMS

Changes in cognitive function

Schizophrenia affects how the thinking part of the brain works, known as cognitive function. These changes can be subtle or obvious, and can affect a person's ability to:

· pay attention, concentrate and remember
· interpret their environment
· use reason and judgment
· understand and process information
· express themselves through language
· read social signals and make sense of social interactions
· plan and organize tasks.

Schizophrenia's effect on thinking can affect the person's ability to work or learn, to follow through on activities of daily living, and to interact in social situations. Cognitive symptoms can be challenging because they tend to be long-lasting and may not respond to medications.

> *I don't feel like I've improved since I've been on medi-cation. I feel like I've stayed the same. My thoughts are not as jumbled, but my life hasn't improved. I'm still struggling with everyday living. Just going shopping, cooking my meals.* — Ann

Disturbances of feeling or mood

Many of the symptoms of schizophrenia can make it hard for a person to identify and express their feelings. At times they may have inappropriate or intense bursts of feeling that seem to come out of nowhere, while at other times they may feel empty of emotions.

People with schizophrenia may also experience depression, sometimes with thoughts of suicide (suicide is discussed in more detail on page 18). Anxiety may also occur, especially if the person is feeling distress as a result of their symptoms. Some may also feel anger.

Ambivalence

Ambivalence means having conflicting ideas, wishes and feelings toward a person, thing or situation. A person with schizophrenia may feel uncertainty and doubt. It may be hard for them to make up their mind about anything, even common decisions such as what to wear in the morning. Often, even when they are able to make a decision, they find it hard to stick with it.

Lack of insight

People with schizophrenia may not consider what they are experiencing to be an illness. This lack of insight or awareness may be present throughout the illness, and can contribute to a decision to reject a recommended treatment plan. Family members may find this particularly difficult to understand and accept.

> The first time I went to the hospital, the cops put me in an ambulance. I was a different person the next day, but I didn't accept the diagnosis and I didn't accept medications when I left the hospital a week later. — Moshe

How is schizophrenia diagnosed?

There is no lab test, scan or physical exam that can be used to diagnose schizophrenia. However, these types of investigations can be used to rule out other medical conditions with similar symptoms.

A diagnosis can be made by any physician. However, it is best made by a psychiatrist or psychologist, as these mental health specialists have specific training and experience in assessing, diagnosing and treating schizophrenia. Psychologists can assess, diagnose and provide psychotherapy for mental health disorders, but medication can only be prescribed by psychiatrists and other physicians.

To arrive at a diagnosis, the physician or psychologist asks structured questions about how the person is thinking and behaving. This information gathering, called an assessment, may be completed in one meeting or may involve several meetings. The clinician may also gather information from family members or others who are familiar with the person's history. Other clinicians, such as social workers, nurses or occupational therapists, may also help to collect information.

A diagnosis of schizophrenia is based on:
· the information gathered
· ruling out other possible explanations
· the physician or psychologist's clinical judgment
· certain symptoms, described above, that have been present for at least one month and last for at least six months
· symptoms that are severe enough to have an impact on the person's social, educational or occupational functioning and abilities.

The type and severity of symptoms can vary among people with a diagnosis of schizophrenia.

Arriving at a diagnosis can be challenging as there are other related disorders that share some features with schizophrenia (e.g., hallucinations and delusions) while also having important differences. Schizophrenia is now considered to be part of a spectrum of psychological disorders that feature psychosis. There are also medical problems that can cause similar symptoms. The expertise of a physician or psychologist is crucial to arriving at an accurate diagnosis. Some of the disorders related to schizophrenia (or with similar symptoms) are:

- schizoaffective disorder
- delusional disorder
- schizophreniform disorder
- bipolar disorder
- depression with psychosis
- schizotypal personality disorder
- substance-induced psychosis
- brief psychotic disorder.

Research has shown that the earlier a person can get a correct diagnosis and treatment for schizophrenia, the better the long-term outcome. Family involvement and advocacy can help ensure that the person gets access to a diagnosis and care as soon as possible.

The GP didn't even have a clue. The psychiatrist said it was addiction. There was no attempt at a mental health diagnosis. It took two years. — Gilda

It got so chaotic, and I totally lost it. I had a nervous breakdown, and they diagnosed me with schizoaffective disorder and I don't know why, I'm not sure, but I know my thoughts were chaotic, I was paranoid, and I was extremely anxious, I was wound up, my stress level was high. — Ann

There was a family history so when I noticed there were changes I sought help. I do think being able to recognize the signs and getting treatment in the early stages helped. I was able to get a degree, to hold a job and have friends and live on my own. — S

Co-occurring issues

People with schizophrenia often have other issues at the same time. These may include physical health problems, substance use or a history of traumatic events in their lives. Even on its own, recovery from schizophrenia can be a significant challenge for the person with the illness and their family. When these co-occurring issues are present, their treatment should be integrated into the overall recovery plan.

PHYSICAL HEALTH

In general, people with schizophrenia have poorer health and are at higher risk for premature death than the overall population. The most common cause of death is cardiovascular disease. This is partly due to lifestyle factors such as obesity, smoking, diabetes, high blood pressure and high cholesterol. Additionally, some of the medications used to treat schizophrenia can cause weight gain or worsen other risk factors, which can lead to diabetes and other serious health problems.

People with schizophrenia have a harder time accessing health care services, and their physical health issues often don't get proper medical attention. For people with any mental health disorder, regular exercise, a healthy diet and regular visits with a primary health care provider are essential to overall health, wellness and recovery.

SUBSTANCE USE AND SMOKING

There is no simple explanation why substance use and smoking are more common in people with schizophrenia. Research suggests that substance use may increase the chance of developing schizophrenia, and also that schizophrenia may increase the chance of developing a substance use disorder. In addition, certain people may have a genetic vulnerability that increases the chance of developing both schizophrenia and a substance use disorder. More research is needed to understand the link.

People with schizophrenia may use substances to:
· "self-medicate" (relieve symptoms or distress)
· relax, increase pleasure, fight boredom or make social connections
· cope with past trauma, poverty, social isolation, homelessness and stigma.

The relationship between substance use problems and schizophrenia is complicated and important. For example:
· Smoking cigarettes contributes to poor physical health outcomes in people with schizophrenia.
· Nicotine may interact with some antipsychotic medications and reduce their effectiveness.
· Cannabis use at an early age may increase the risk of developing schizophrenia.

Substance use by people with schizophrenia can:
· have a negative impact on relationships, employment, finances and physical health
· lead to legal problems
· worsen psychotic symptoms
· worsen depression and anxiety
· reduce the effectiveness of medication and psychosocial treatments
· increase the risk of relapse, hospitalization, housing problems, disruptive behaviour and relationship problems.

Despite the many negative consequences of substance use, a person may still feel that substance use helps them in some way. They may not be ready or willing to reduce or quit their substance use. However, they may be open to considering ways to reduce the harm of their use (e.g., where they use, how they use, who they use with). This kind of approach can help to start conversations about substance use, and help people to move toward reducing or stopping their use.

The best approach to helping people with schizophrenia quit or make changes to their substance use, including smoking, is one that recognizes the relationship between schizophrenia and substance use. These specialized "concurrent disorders" treatment services are not widely available, however, and can be difficult to find.

TRAUMA

Childhood trauma, in particular childhood sexual abuse, may increase the risk that schizophrenia will develop in a person who has other risk factors for the illness. (Risk factors are described in chapter 2.)

For some people with schizophrenia, the experience of acute psychosis (e.g., hearing voices, believing that others are out to harm them) and being hospitalized can be traumatic in itself.

The connection between psychological trauma and schizophrenia is not fully understood. But it is known that the effects of trauma—particularly traumas early in life—can complicate recovery. The best approach to assessment, recovery planning and all aspects of care considers trauma and its impacts. This is referred to as "trauma-informed" care.

POVERTY

Poverty increases the risk of schizophrenia, and schizophrenia increases the risk of poverty. Poverty can have a negative impact on mental and physical health. Adequate housing, employment and financial and social support can help to protect people with schizophrenia from the negative effects of poverty.

STIGMA

Public attitudes, stereotypes and beliefs about schizophrenia can cause stigma—that is, negative and inaccurate beliefs that can have a profound impact on those living with the illness. Common beliefs—that people with schizophrenia are dangerous and violent, or that they are irresponsible and lazy—have a negative impact on individuals' work, housing and social opportunities. Stigma is mostly a result of people misunderstanding schizophrenia.

When people with schizophrenia are negatively and inaccurately judged by others, they can come to believe these negative things about themselves. This can lead to hopelessness, helplessness and a negative self-image, which can hinder recovery.

There are strategies that can help people with schizophrenia and their families to cope with and combat stigma. They include:
· developing a recovery plan
· connecting with peers and family
· maintaining a sense of hope for the future
· educating oneself and others about schizophrenia
· challenging negative beliefs about oneself
· critically reviewing information about schizophrenia portrayed in the media, and encouraging others to do the same
· getting involved in anti-stigma initiatives, such as those led by the Schizophrenia Society, the Canadian Mental Health Association (CMHA) and the Mental Health Commission of Canada.

Combatting stigma is an important way to support the recovery of people with schizophrenia.

People should understand that schizophrenia could happen to anybody. Mental illness doesn't discriminate, people do. — Moshe

There's a sense of self-denial because there's a lot of stigma attached to it, and misconceptions about what it is. People don't want to identify themselves as having it. They're like, that's not me. — S

Schizophrenia and violence

VIOLENCE TOWARD OTHERS

A common myth about people with schizophrenia is that they are violent. In fact, people with schizophrenia are more often the victims of violent crime than they are the perpetrators. Homelessness, substance use and severe symptoms increase the risk that a person with schizophrenia will be victimized.

Aggression and hostility *can* be associated with schizophrenia, though spontaneous or random assault by a person with schizophrenia is rare. It is not possible to predict with certainty who may be violent. However, factors that can increase the risk include:

· a history of violence
· substance use
· not participating in a treatment and recovery plan (e.g., not taking medications)
· impulsivity (tending to act without thinking about the consequences)
· being a younger male
· previous involvement with the criminal justice system.

It is rare, but some people with schizophrenia experience auditory hallucinations that command them to harm others, or delusional beliefs that compel them to protect themselves through violence. Having these types of hallucinations or delusions does not mean that a person will act on them. If you or someone you know is experiencing symptoms that command or compel violence, get help from a health care provider right away.

SUICIDE

People with schizophrenia are six times more likely to attempt suicide than the general population. However, this does not mean that a diagnosis of schizophrenia will lead to suicidal behaviour or death by suicide. There are particular risk factors for suicide, including:

- a history of suicidal thoughts or attempts
- positive symptoms (delusions, hallucinations, disorganization of thought, speech or behaviour)
- co-occurring depression or substance abuse
- lack of insight and awareness of schizophrenia's effect on one's mental state
- lack of treatment or downgrading of the level of care
- negative beliefs about medications; not taking medications as prescribed
- chronic pain or illness
- hopelessness
- a family history of suicide
- social isolation or limited external supports
- agitation and impulsivity
- childhood psychological trauma.

People with schizophrenia may require extra support, attention and treatment due to increased risk of suicide when:

- the person is experiencing active and intense psychotic symptoms
- the person is very depressed

· the illness is in its early stages
· the person has been discharged from hospital.

People experiencing suicidal thoughts may attempt to hurt themselves. Suicidal thoughts should be taken seriously and should always be discussed with a health professional or therapist. In the event of an emergency, contact 911 or go to your nearest emergency room. Family members may need support and assistance to cope effectively in such situations.

2 What causes schizophrenia?

We don't know if it's cannabis, if it's stress, if it's bio-logical, or trauma—all those impact it. There's no definitive answer. For me it was stress. I felt a lot of guilt and shame about the way I ended a relationship. I also felt like I was failing in other areas of my life. I feel I created a spiritual fantasy to find a sense of meaning and significance in my life. — Moshe

It is not known for certain what causes schizophrenia, but like most other mental health problems, researchers believe that a combination of biological and environmental factors contribute to its development.

Because the specific causes of schizophrenia are still unknown, we cannot predict who will get it. However, researchers have dis-covered that certain factors increase the risk of a person developing schizophrenia. These risk factors are described below.

Biological theories

Biological theories of the causes of schizophrenia suggest that:
· Genetics plays a role—the risk of developing schizophrenia is higher when a close family member has the illness.

- The symptoms of schizophrenia result from an imbalance of brain chemicals (e.g., the neurotransmitters dopamine and glutamate).
- Structural differences in the brains of people with schizophrenia have been discovered; however, it is not known if these differences are the cause of schizophrenia or if schizophrenia causes the differences.
- Current research suggests that schizophrenia may be influenced by brain development factors before and around the time of birth, and during childhood and adolescence. These different influences are thought to set the stage for schizophrenia, which usually appears in late adolescence or early adulthood.

Environmental theories

Environmental factors are those that exist outside of a person's body, in their surroundings. Biological factors, such as having a family member with schizophrenia, have long been recognized as important. However, we now know that the picture is more complex. Stressful life events and other environmental factors increase the risk that someone with genetic vulnerability will develop the illness. Research into the role of environmental factors suggests that:

- People who have experienced social hardship or trauma, particularly during childhood (e.g., sexual abuse or lengthy separation from parents), have a higher risk of developing schizophrenia.
- Cannabis use increases the risk of developing schizophrenia in youth and of triggering an earlier onset of the illness in people who are genetically vulnerable.
- Being born or spending one's childhood in an urban environment, rather than a rural one, increases the risk of developing schizophrenia. This may be due to environmental factors such as social isolation and overcrowding.

· Particular immigrant and refugee groups in Ontario may have a higher risk of developing psychotic disorders. As more research is being done, similar findings are emerging internationally.

Exactly how these risk factors interact to cause schizophrenia is not yet fully understood. The presence of one or more of these factors does not mean that schizophrenia will develop. Rather than being caused by a single factor, schizophrenia appears to be influenced by biological and environmental factors that interact in complex ways. As research continues into the causes of the illness, other ways to diagnose and treat it may be revealed.

> *I wish people understood that it's not the person's fault that they are sick. If I could not be sick, I would choose not to be.* — Ann

3 Treatments for schizophrenia

There are two halves to the treatment equation: the medication, and the other half, people, social settings, introspection and reflection, goal setting—the practical stuff. For me, the medication was necessary, especially in the beginning. There was a lot going on inside my head and the medication helped to slow down my thoughts. It gave me a chance to rebuild my life. — Moshe

Treatment for schizophrenia often begins with medication. Psychosocial supports, such as psychotherapy, education and peer support, can also promote recovery. Treatment needs to address other health concerns, too—regular check-ups with a family doctor are important.

Families can play an important role in a person's recovery. Family counselling can help people with schizophrenia and their families to understand and manage challenges related to the illness.

Understanding the treatments and supports offered will allow you to discuss them with your treatment team, and to develop your own recovery plan.

The treatment team

The treatment team can include nurses, doctors (including psychiatrists), social workers, psychologists, pharmacists, occupational therapists, recreational therapists, dieticians, peer support workers and spiritual advisors. The role of the treatment team is to help you build a recovery plan. A collaborative, trusting relationship with the team members can help you to recover your health and re-engage with things that are meaningful to you.

Medication

The main medications used to treat symptoms of schizophrenia are antipsychotics. They are often used in combination with medications for other mental health symptoms, such as mood stabilizers, sedatives and antidepressants,[1] and medications to help with the side-effects of antipsychotics.

Antipsychotics (previously called neuroleptics) can reduce or relieve symptoms of psychosis, such as hallucinations and delusions. In a person with acute psychosis, these medications can help to control symptoms and to calm and clear confusion within hours or days, but can take up to six weeks to reach their full effect. Over a longer term, antipsychotics can help to prevent further episodes of psychosis.

While they can help most people with schizophrenia, antipsychotics can have serious side-effects. The aim of medication treatment is to reduce and control symptoms while keeping side-effects at a minimum.

---

[1] Further information about these types of medications can be found online at www.camh.ca/en/hospital/health_information/a_z_mental_health_and_addiction_information.

WHAT DO ANTIPSYCHOTICS DO?

Psychosis is believed to be caused in part by overactivity of a brain chemical called dopamine. Antipsychotics work by blocking this dopamine effect. This helps to relieve the positive symptoms of psychosis, but it does not always make them go away completely. A person may still hear voices and have delusions, but they are more able to recognize what isn't real and to focus on other things, such as work, school or family.

> *Some members of my family think that when I'm on medication, I should be 100 per cent normal, which is not true. The medication doesn't cure all the symptoms.*
> — Moustafa

TYPES OF ANTIPSYCHOTICS

Antipsychotic medications are generally divided into categories: first-generation (also called typical antipsychotics) and the newer second- and third-generation (atypical).

The newer, second-generation (atypical) antipsychotics include clozapine (Clozaril),[2] olanzapine (Zyprexa), quetiapine (Seroquel), risperidone (Risperdal), paliperidone (Invega), ziprasidone (Zeldox), lurasidone (Latuda) and asenapine (Saphris). Aripiprazole (Abilify) is classified as a third-generation (atypical) antipsychotic.

The first generation (typical) antipsychotics that are commonly used include chlorpromazine, flupenthixol, fluphenazine, haloperidol, loxapine, perphenazine, pimozide, thiothixene, trifluoperazine and zuclopenthixol.

2 Medications are referred to in two ways: by their generic name and by their brand or trade name. Brand names available in Canada appear here in brackets. Older medications are generally referred to by their generic name.

The newer and older medications work equally well overall, although no drug or type of drug works equally well for everyone who takes it. You may need to try different antipsychotics before finding the one that works best for you.

Clozapine often works even when other medications have failed. However, it is not the first choice for treatment because it requires monitoring of white blood cell counts.

HOW ARE ANTIPSYCHOTICS TAKEN?

Most of these medications are given in tablet form, some are liquids and others are given as injections. Some are available as long-lasting ("depot") injections, which may be given anywhere from once a week to once a month.

Treatment begins with a low dose; your response to the medication is monitored closely for any side-effects.

Using substances—including alcohol or tobacco—while taking antipsychotic medication can interfere with the treatment and may make symptoms worse.

SIDE-EFFECTS

Some people experience no side-effects. If they do occur, they may be noticed within hours, days or weeks of starting treatment. Side-effects vary depending on the medication and on the person taking it. Common side-effects include fatigue, sedation, dizziness, dry mouth, blurry vision and constipation. Though they are bothersome, most side-effects are not serious, and diminish over time.

Some people accept the side-effects as a trade-off for the relief these medications can bring. Others find them distressing and may choose to speak to their physician about other medication options. Your physician may prescribe a lower dose, add a medication to reduce the side-effects, or recommend a different medication altogether.

If you are troubled by side-effects that are tolerable, continue to take your medication as prescribed and let your physician know as soon as possible. If the side-effects are not tolerable, go to your nearest emergency room.

Treatment with antipsychotics does carry a risk of some more severe side-effects that can affect your physical health. Your physician will check for signs of the following effects at your regular follow-up visits, and treatment can be adjusted. Most side-effects can be minimized with other medications. Changing your medication can also help. Be sure to talk to your doctor about any side-effects you experience.

Movement effects
Some people experience tremors, muscle stiffness and tics. Usually, the higher the dose, the more severe these effects are. The risk of movement effects (also called extrapyramidal effects) may be lower with the second-generation medications than with the older drugs. Other drugs (e.g., benztropine [Cogentin]) can be used to control the movement effects.

Dizziness
Dizziness may occur, especially when getting up from a sitting or lying position, because of temporary lowered blood pressure. Getting up slowly can help prevent dizziness.

Cardiac arrhythmias
Some medications can cause arrhythmias, where the heart beats too fast, too slow or with an irregular rhythm. Cardiac arrhythmias can increase the risk of heart disease.

Weight gain

It is not yet fully understood why people who take antipsychotics put on weight. Whatever the cause, weight gain can increase a person's risk of diabetes and heart disease. These effects are known as metabolic effects. A healthy diet and regular exercise can help to limit weight gain.

Diabetes

Schizophrenia is a risk factor for diabetes. Antipsychotic drugs can increase this risk.

Agitation and sedation

Antipsychotics make some people feel agitated, or "wired," and unable to stop moving. This side-effect is called akathisia, and may be mistaken for a worsening of the illness. For some people antipsychotics can have the opposite effect, making them sedated or tired. Some people may feel both wired and tired at the same time.

Tardive dyskinesia

Tardive dyskinesia (TD) is a condition that causes people to have repetitive involuntary movements of the tongue, lips, jaw or fingers. The risk of TD is highest with first-generation antipsychotics, although it can occur with the newer drugs as well. If TD does develop, there are ways to identify it at an early stage and to modify treatment. This will reduce the risk that the condition will continue or worsen.

Hormonal and sexual side-effects

Some antipsychotics can cause changes in sex drive, along with other sexual problems, menstrual changes, and the abnormal production of breast milk (in both men and women).

Neuroleptic malignant syndrome

This is a rare but serious complication. Signs include fever, muscle stiffness and delirium (e.g., disorientation and confusion). This condition can be life threatening and requires immediate treatment.

> *Sometimes doctors do not want to change medications if they perceive you as stable, but sometimes finding the right medication for you outweighs not changing. I had a lot of side-effects: weight gain, stiffness and muscle movement from TD; it was pretty bad. Changing the medication helped. I needed to find the right med, and I went through several. I knew how I was feeling. I knew me. People have to advocate for themselves.* — S

HOW LONG DO I NEED TO TAKE ANTIPSYCHOTICS?

You will be advised to keep taking antipsychotic medications even after the symptoms are controlled. If you stop taking medication too early, there is a high risk that symptoms will return. This may not happen until several months later.

Continuing to take the medication reduces the risk of relapse, and can reduce the intensity of symptoms if you do have a relapse. Preventing relapse helps to promote recovery and to improve the overall outcome of the illness. Talk with your doctor about how long you should continue taking medication.

> *If I don't take my medication for a couple months, I end up with another episode. I end up in the hospital. That's why I am strictly religious about taking my medications. I'm going to have to take medication for the rest of my life, and I'm okay with that. When I don't take it, I spin out.* — Moustafa

HOW MUCH DO MEDICATIONS COST?

The cost of medications varies, depending on the type. Some or all of the cost may be covered if you qualify for a provincial drug benefit program, or if you have a prescription drug benefit plan through your work or through a family member. Students may have drug benefits through their college or university.

For example, in Ontario, the Ontario Drug Benefit is available to people who:
· are on social assistance (Ontario Works)
· are on disability (Ontario Disability Support Program)
· have a low income (Trillium Drug Program)
· are 65 years of age or older.

Electroconvulsive therapy

When symptoms of schizophrenia are not relieved by medication, or when a person with schizophrenia is severely depressed, electroconvulsive therapy (ECT) may be advised.

ECT does not resemble the shock therapy portrayed in older films and TV shows. Now patients are given a muscle relaxant and a general anesthetic before a mild electrical current is applied to one or both sides of the brain. The person being treated shows little visible movement. A course of ECT consists of a number of treatments that most often are given three times a week. The total number of treatments, and how often they are given, is decided in consultation with a physician.

Some people may experience side-effects of ECT, such as a headache or jaw pain when they wakeup after the treatment. This usually requires only a mild painkiller such as acetaminophen (Tylenol).

Some loss of recent memory or problems with concentration usually occurs during treatment. These symptoms improve over a few weeks after the course of ECT is finished. Some people report memory problems *after* ECT treatment has been completed, but these problems usually improve within a few weeks or months.

Transcranial magnetic stimulation

Transcranial magnetic stimulation (TMS) is a newer form of treatment that applies magnetic waves to the brain to stimulate nerve cells. This treatment would be considered in addition to medication. Researchers are still exploring its effectiveness.

Psychosocial therapies and supports

Psychosocial therapies and supports help people to develop recovery skills, such as setting and achieving goals (e.g., improving self-care, pursuing education, finding or changing a job). The choice of therapies and supports will depend on your unique needs and on what is available in your community.

PSYCHOEDUCATION

Psychoeducation provides information to help people deal with a mental health condition, such as how to manage symptoms and medication side-effects, and how to prevent relapse. It also provides information on the recovery process, such as how to maintain a sense of well-being and how to develop skills to manage stress and solve problems. Psychoeducation can be offered individually or in groups, and may be tailored to the person with a mental health condition or to family members and friends.

THERAPIES

Several effective psychosocial therapies for schizophrenia, in individual or group format, are now available to complement treatment with medication. Group therapy can allow you to learn about other people's experiences with the illness, which can help to reduce isolation and promote recovery. Discuss your needs with your service providers to determine which kind of therapy is best for you.

Cognitive-behavioural therapy for psychosis

The way you think about a situation can affect how you feel and how you behave. Cognitive-behavioural therapy for psychosis (CBT-p) explores the connection between your thoughts, feelings and behaviours and your experience of the symptoms of schizophrenia. CBT-p can help you to better manage your symptoms and stress, to understand the impact of the illness on your life, and to recognize how alcohol and other substance use affects symptoms. For some people, CBT-p helps to reduce symptoms and prevent relapse.

Cognitive adaptation training

People with schizophrenia may have cognitive symptoms that affect their ability to remember, focus, pay attention and solve problems. These symptoms can make it hard to carry out everyday functions, such as taking medication and self-care. Cognitive adaptation training (CAT) uses individually customized supports, such as signs and checklists, to help people manage their daily tasks. Clinicians who provide CAT help clients to:
· identify barriers to their goals
· organize their living space
· set up and practice new routines
· use different types of prompts and reminders.

The goal of this training is to help people with schizophrenia live more independently and to achieve their life goals.

Concurrent disorders treatment

Mental health and substance use issues often occur together. When they do, they are often closely related and affect each other. For this reason, treatment for these co-occurring issues (also called concurrent disorders) is most effective when it addresses both issues at the same time. Concurrent disorders treatment may include counselling, education about substances and the impact of substance use on symptoms, medication management, stress management and relapse prevention. It may also include support in other life areas, such as housing and employment.

Family therapy and supports

Having a supportive family can be a huge help to people with schizophrenia. However, family members themselves often experience significant stress. This can make it harder for them to be supportive and to take care of themselves. Individual and family counselling, psychoeducation workshops and support groups can help people to develop coping strategies and effective communication skills, which allow them to better support the family member and to practice self-care. (See chapter 6 for more information about family supports.)

Peer support

Peer support workers are people with lived experience of a mental health condition who are trained to provide support that is based on empathy and understanding. Having gone through their own personal recovery, peer support workers are able to help you plan and move through the steps of your own recovery. Support focuses on your strengths, rather than the illness, and on self-empowerment, self-advocacy and promoting hope. Peer support workers are important members of the treatment team. Peer support may be available one-on-one or in groups.

Complementary approaches

You may wish to add other approaches to conventional treatments. Examples of complementary approaches include herbal medicine, acupuncture, homeopathy, naturopathy, meditation, yoga, Ayurveda (an ancient medical system from India), nutritional supplements and vitamins. However, none of these approaches has been tested to determine the effect on the symptoms of schizophrenia. Check with your treatment team about any complementary or alternative therapies you are taking or thinking about trying—especially herbal medicine or vitamins, which may interfere with the effectiveness of medications.

Medical care, physical activity and diet

Important ways to manage health problems and to achieve and maintain physical health include:
· regular visits to a family doctor or specialist for medical care
· physical activity
· a healthy diet.

Physical activity positively affects both physical and mental health. Choose any physical activity you enjoy, and adapt it to your fitness level and to any medication side-effects you may experience. A healthy diet can help you manage the health problems often associated with schizophrenia. Look to your family doctor, a dietician or other treatment provider for help with planning your diet and exercise routine.

4 Hospital, intensive support and community support

With proper support and medication, schizophrenia may cause few or no interruptions in a person's life. However, a brief time in hospital may be necessary during an active phase of the illness. The goal of admission to hospital is to provide the treatment the person needs to regain their health and return home as soon as possible.

While the person is in hospital, families can play an important role in helping their relative and the treatment team to plan for discharge (leaving the hospital) and beyond. When the person with schizophrenia returns home, intensive and community supports may be available, if needed. These can help the person to make the transition back to the community and provide on-going support.

Hospitalization

People with schizophrenia may need to be admitted to hospital at times—for example, if the person is aggressive or suicidal or is not looking after their own basic needs.

VOLUNTARY AND INVOLUNTARY ADMISSION

Patients may be admitted to hospital *voluntarily*. This means that they:
· agree to enter the hospital, and
· are free to leave at any time.

The law also allows any doctor to admit a person to hospital *involuntarily*. This means the person may not agree that he or she needs help, and does not want to be in the hospital. This can happen if the doctor has assessed the person and believes there is a serious risk that the person:
· will physically harm himself or herself, or
· will physically harm someone else, or
· has shown or is showing lack of competence to care for himself or herself.

If no doctor has seen the person, families also may ask a justice of the peace (a local public officer with legal authority) to order a psychiatric assessment. They must provide convincing evidence that the person's illness is a danger to himself or herself or to others. The police are sometimes needed to help to get a person to hospital.

Laws protect the rights of people who are admitted involuntarily. For instance, a rights advisor will visit. The rights advisor will ensure that if the person wishes, he or she has the chance to appeal the involuntary status before an independent board of lawyers, doctors and laypeople.

For more information about mental health laws and patient rights in Ontario, see the website of the Psychiatric Patient Advocate Office www.sse.gov.on.ca/mohltc/ppao.

INPATIENT TREATMENT

A typical hospital stay may last between a few days and several weeks. During this time, goals and plans for treatment and recovery will be identified.

Patients take part in group educational and therapeutic programs, as well as individual sessions with medical, nursing and other professional staff. Programs and services may vary, depending on the person's needs and location. While the person is in hospital, medications may be changed or doses adjusted. Families may be asked to meet with medical, social work or other staff.

Discharge planning begins as early as possible. Patients can expect to leave the hospital once their symptoms have improved enough that they can safely care for themselves at home, and when ongoing treatment and support has been arranged.

Intensive supports in the community

In Ontario, intensive supports include assertive community treatment (ACT) teams and intensive case management (ICM). Both work closely with the person with schizophrenia to create a recovery plan, to provide outreach, and to co-ordinate services to help the person work toward their goals. Each person's goals will be different, but they can include improving housing conditions, managing physical health (e.g., weight loss, diabetes care), building coping skills, managing substance use issues, creating healthy social relationships, and returning to school or work. Intensive supports may also be provided through a community treatment order (CTO).

ASSERTIVE COMMUNITY TREATMENT TEAMS

An ACT team helps to support the person with schizophrenia with day-to-day living. Teams are usually either linked to a hospital or run through a community agency that is linked to a nearby hospital. The team may include a psychiatrist, peer support worker, registered nurse, social worker, occupational therapist, addiction specialist and vocational specialist.

ACT teams provide intensive support and co-ordinate services for people living with serious and ongoing mental health issues. This usually means people who have been hospitalized multiple times, and who may need a high level of support to manage living in the community. ACT team members often meet with clients several times a week, for example, in the client's home, a family doctor's office or a community centre. ACT services aim to promote consistent, ongoing support over a long period.

Patients who need support in the community and who meet other criteria may be referred to an ACT team by their treatment team. The local office of the CMHA or another mental health agency can tell you more about ACT teams in your community. ACT teams are more common in larger cities.

INTENSIVE CASE MANAGEMENT

ICM is similar to the support provided by ACT teams. The difference is that instead of a team, support is usually provided by an individual case manager (e.g., a nurse, social worker or occupational therapist). Case managers see their clients regularly and help to co-ordinate care and services.

COMMUNITY TREATMENT ORDER

A CTO is a legal agreement between a physician and a person with a serious mental illness, or the person's substitute decision maker.[1] A CTO is for people who have been in hospital several times, and have benefited from the treatment, but do not continue their treatment after leaving hospital. A CTO sets conditions and provides services that allow the person to receive care and support in the community, rather than in a hospital. If you are a substitute decision maker and you believe your family member would benefit from a CTO, talk to the person's care team.

Community supports

Programs may be available to help people with schizophrenia live in their own community. The kinds of services offered vary with location, but can include financial, housing, education, employment and social support. The Schizophrenia Society and CMHA keep lists of local programs (e.g., peer support or consumer/survivor initiatives, drop-ins or support groups.) Your treatment team can also help to connect you to the supports you need.

Community supports can be anything from support groups (where people with similar life experiences meet and support each other) to places to go in a crisis. Below you'll find some information about a few types of community support.

CONSUMER/SURVIVOR INITIATIVES

People who have used mental health services sometimes choose

---

[1] When a doctor determines that a person is incapable of making decisions about their own care, a family member (or a public guardian or trustee) may be appointed as a substitute decision maker.

to identify themselves as consumer/survivors (consumers of mental health services and survivors either of their personal mental health issue or of the mental health system—depending on their experience).

Consumer/survivor initiatives are run by and for people who have lived experience (past or current) with the mental health system. These programs were developed as an alternative to traditional mental health services provided by hospitals or community mental health agencies. They offer education, information and support, and often also provide social/recreational opportunities, as well as work/employment opportunities with businesses run by consumer/survivors.

CLUBHOUSES

Clubhouses are local community centres for people living with mental health issues. Members develop skills and work closely with peers and support staff to run the daily operations of the clubhouse. They prepare meals, build social connections, create newsletters, track members' participation and more. Clubhouses also offer support to help people transition into employment. Clubhouses differ from traditional mental health services in that consumer/survivors partner with staff to run the clubhouse, rather than simply receiving services from staff.

SUPPORTED EMPLOYMENT / SUPPORTED EDUCATION PROGRAMS

Employment programs support your goal to return to work. They can help you to rebuild your work skills, to build self-confidence and to find jobs that fit your abilities and needs. These programs offer services such as job assessment, career counselling, aptitude testing, job search skills and on-the-job training.

Supported education programs support your goal to return to school with in-class training and skill-building. They are typically offered through community colleges, and mix academic upgrading classes with skills-based classes such as assertiveness training, communication and stress management.

Skills training programs are offered through community colleges, universities, high school upgrading programs, libraries and community centres. These programs work on specific skills (e.g., computer training) as a step toward employment.

DROP-IN CENTRES

Drop-in centres focus on providing recreational and social opportunities rather than employment opportunities. They may have a structured schedule of recreation, meals and educational sessions, and are typically open to anyone. They can also be used as a place to rest, meet up with friends, or use a phone, computer, shower or laundry equipment. Drop-in centres can often help link you with other community supports.

SUPPORT GROUPS

Self-help groups (also known as mutual aid or peer support groups) are made up of people who have a common concern, such as a mental health issue. These groups are usually led by people with lived experience of mental health problems and are open-ended, so you can join or leave at any time. Group members meet to give and receive support, and to exchange coping and problem-solving strategies and other information. Support groups help members to feel connected through sharing their experiences with others who can understand what they are going through.

5 Recovery and relapse prevention

Recovery to me means not putting limitations on myself.
To feel I can achieve things. What really worked for
me is setting goals. I like to make lists of possibilities. It
helps you get back into life. — S

What is recovery?

Psychiatry has changed over time, and so has the expected role of people receiving mental health services. Historically, it was thought that schizophrenia was a chronic and deteriorating condition and that people needed to be looked after, often in institutions, for the rest of their lives. This way of thinking has shifted.

In the late 1980s, a new way of thinking about recovery emerged from research evidence and the advocacy work of people with lived experience of schizophrenia. Recovery was now seen as a process of gaining control over one's life and finding meaning, rather than as the total absence of symptoms. People with schizophrenia could now expect to be involved in planning their own treatment and making decisions about their lives. They could expect to live in the community and to have meaningful lives.

This concept of recovery is now a guiding principle of mental health care.

The process of recovery

Recovery is often described as a journey. It is not a straight line from sick to well, but a winding road that follows an individual's experience, including bumps, curves, potholes and smooth sailing. Each person's recovery is unique.

The following five key recovery processes, known as CHIME, were identified from personal recovery stories. Recovery may be seen as moving toward these conditions, rather than being free from symptoms.

- **Connectedness:** Having meaningful social connections, supportive relationships, peer support and being part of a community
- **Hope and optimism for the future:** Having aspirations, dreams and beliefs that recovery is possible; having motivation to change
- **Identity:** Having a positive sense of self and overcoming experiences of stigma
- **Meaning in life:** Having roles, experiences, goals and personal values that bring meaning to your life (e.g., through spirituality, work, education or relationships)
- **Empowerment:** Recognizing your own strengths and having ownership, responsibility and control over your own life (Leamy et al., 2011)

> *If a person is not harming themselves or others, then who am I to say what is right for that person? In that context, recovery can mean anything to anybody. It's up to the person.* — Moshe

Promoting wellness and preventing relapse

Everyone with a serious health problem needs to pay attention to their health, find strategies to maintain health, and prepare for possible relapse (the return of active symptoms). The following strategies can help to promote and maintain wellness for people with schizophrenia:

- **Become an expert on schizophrenia.** Learn about the symptoms, potential treatments and outcomes. Figure out what works for you; this will usually include medication and other support. The websites and other resources listed on page 68 offer information on a variety of schizophrenia-related topics. Consider also asking your service provider to recommend books, support groups or classes that might interest you.

- **Maintain social connections and prevent isolation.** We all need people in our lives who know and care about us. People with schizophrenia sometimes experience symptoms that lead them to become cut off from others. It's important to try to maintain your connections, and to be a part of a community. Besides providing enjoyment, friends may also be able to let you know if they notice changes in your behaviour that could be an early warning sign of relapse. Consider participating in community groups (e.g., cultural, spiritual, religious, special interest) that are meaningful to you.

- **Establish a healthy and active lifestyle.** Eating regular meals and following a balanced, nutritious diet is one of the best ways to take care of yourself. Another is being active. Run, walk, go to the gym, dance or play a sport. Find something that gets you moving that you enjoy. Ask your health care team to help connect you with resources such as dieticians and food services, if needed (e.g., food banks, free meals or community kitchen programs) and options for free or low-cost physical activity.

· **Get the right amount of sleep.** If you feel you are not getting enough sleep, or that you are sleeping too much, talk to your psychiatrist, family doctor or case manager about education and treatment options for improving your sleep.

· **Reduce or stop substance use.** Consider the role that alcohol and other drugs play in your life, and how they affect your mental and physical health and social relationships. Substance use can make it harder to reach recovery goals and to achieve and maintain wellness. Look to your treatment team for help with addressing substance use issues.

· **Establish a medication plan that works for you.** With schizophrenia, maintaining wellness and reaching your recovery goals can depend on taking medications for a long time. Work with your doctor to find the smallest dose of medication to help control your symptoms with the fewest side-effects. This can be on ongoing process, as your needs may change over time. Take your medications as prescribed and work closely with your prescribing doctor to make adjustments as needed.

· **Develop a wellness plan.** Having a personal plan for maintaining your health is an important way of planning your recovery. Consider these actions when developing your wellness plan:
  - Participate in a WRAP group. WRAP stands for Wellness Recovery Action Plan. WRAP groups are peer-led, which means that the leader, as well as the members, has lived experience of mental health challenges. The leader is trained to help the group members develop an individual wellness plan. Your WRAP might include lists of wellness tools, triggers, early

warning signs and signs of relapse, and also a daily wellness plan and crisis plan.

- Collaborate with members of your health care team, such as your family doctor, psychiatrist, peer support worker, case worker and others. They can contribute to your plan by giving input on, for example, the use of medication for treating symptoms and the use of specific therapies.
- Establish advance directives. Advance directives are instructions to your treatment team that you make when you are well, to let them know your preferences and expectations for treatment if you become unwell. Talk with anyone on your health care team about establishing advance directives.

I've taken the Wellness Recovery Action Plan program, and now I facilitate it. It has five key concepts of recovery, and one of them is support. There's also hope, education, personal responsibility and self-advocacy. It's not possible to recover without support. — Moshe

Practical aspects of recovery

HOW MUCH SHOULD I SAY ABOUT MY DIAGNOSIS TO FRIENDS, FAMILY AND OTHER PEOPLE?

It's up to you how much information to disclose about your personal health to your friends, family or anyone else. If you are having trouble explaining schizophrenia, or aren't sure what to say, you can direct them to this booklet, or to online resources (see websites listed on page 68).

WILL I BE ABLE TO WORK OR GO TO SCHOOL?

It is possible that you will be able to attend work or school. However, some symptoms of schizophrenia may affect the way you think, understand and attend to information, so school or work may be interrupted. It can take time to adjust to a new treatment routine, and you may need to learn new skills or strategies to manage tasks that were previously easy. If your symptoms cause interruptions to work or school, you can get help from an occupational therapist (OT), the student accessibility centre at your school, or occupational health supports at work. An OT can help you identify your strengths and develop strategies to address difficulties you may be experiencing, so you can succeed at work or school.

If you receive income supports through social assistance or disability (e.g., the Ontario Disability Support Program), or if you've simply been out of work or school for a long period and would like to return, a variety of resources and programs are available. You can access most programs by connecting with someone from the social assistance program, visiting a local employment support agency, or speaking to someone on your health care team.

See Chapter 4 for information about employment, educational and other types of community supports for people with schizophrenia.

> *People say to me, is she working? Is she going to school?*
> *I had those same expectations. I thought, medication,*
> *good, everything is great, fast forward: can we go to*
> *school again? Nope. We think that once you get the*
> *medication sorted, you're good now. You start expect-*
> *ing things. You have to adjust your expectations. —*
> Gilda

I think it's possible to have a good life despite schizophrenia; to have hope. It's possible to achieve things still. It's not the end of the world. — S

6 Support for family and friends

I'm always thinking that she's going to be okay. I don't think it's a delusion. I think it's good to think that way: to think positive. Never give up hope. — Gilda

A diagnosis of schizophrenia for a loved one can bring many different emotions. Family members[1] and friends may feel loss, guilt, confusion, fear, sadness or anger; some may have all these feelings at once. All these feelings are normal. Lack of knowledge about schizophrenia, and the myths portrayed in the media about the illness, add to these distressing emotions. Learning about the illness and the treatments available, and about how to support and care for your relative while also taking care of your own needs, can help to promote a more positive outlook for everyone.

The way schizophrenia affects a person can vary depending on the person and on the phase of the illness. The effectiveness of treatments can also vary. Some people with schizophrenia will need ongoing support to live in the community; others are able to resume employment and other responsibilities, and can be as independent as anyone. Having family and friends who offer support and respect

---

[1] Although this chapter uses the terms "family," "family member" and "relative," the information can also apply to friends.

can make an important difference in the quality of life for people with schizophrenia, and in helping them to achieve their recovery goals.

The person with schizophrenia still has strengths, talents and abilities, even when the symptoms of the illness conceal these qualities. The symptoms may require treatment, and your family member may require support, but they are still the same person, with hopes and goals for the future.

Confidentiality and legal issues

Family members need a basic understanding of the laws that protect the rights of people with mental illness. For example:
· Privacy laws prevent the health care team from discussing an adult patient's health information with anyone outside the team, including the person's family, unless the patient gives permission.
· Patients have the right to refuse treatment.

Exceptions to these rules include:
· When a person is at risk or harming himself or herself, or others. When risk is involved, the person may be admitted for involuntary treatment for three days.
· When a doctor determines that a person is unable to make decisions about his or her own care. In this situation, a family member or public guardian or trustee may be appointed as a substitute decision maker.

Some laws protecting the rights of mental health patients vary depending on where you live. For more information, talk with your relative's doctor, or check with your local chapter of the CMHA or Schizophrenia Society.

Common concerns

WILL MY FAMILY MEMBER LIVE A PRODUCTIVE AND HAPPY LIFE?

With treatment and support, people with schizophrenia can and do live productive and happy lives. However, the illness can limit a person's functioning, and the recovery process takes time. People with schizophrenia, or any illness, do best when given time to heal. Reducing your relative's stress may help to prevent another active phase of the illness. Daily responsibilities should be increased gradually. Your patience, understanding and support will help your relative to reach their full potential.

WHAT SHOULD I TELL FRIENDS AND RELATIVES?

How much you and your family tell other people about your relative's illness will depend on your own comfort level, and on your relative's wishes. Look for opportunities to educate friends and family about schizophrenia and how it affects your family member. Share this guide, and the resources listed on page 68, and offer to talk about the illness with friends and relatives. When others better understand your family member's experience, it helps to build their compassion and can bring them into your family member's network of support. A wider support network is better for the family member who is ill, and for everyone involved.

WHAT SUPPORTS ARE AVAILABLE TO FAMILIES?

Any type of serious health diagnosis in the family can be stressful, but the stigma often associated with a mental health diagnosis can make it hard to seek out support. If you or your relative does not feel ready to share information about the illness with friends or family, there are many community agencies that offer confidential support and counselling. Family support and education groups are especially recommended if your family member is going through an initial, acute phase of the illness. For information about supports available in your community, talk to your family member's care team, or contact your local chapter of the Schizophrenia Society or CMHA. See page 68 for contact information.

WHAT SHOULD I DO IF MY FAMILY MEMBER DOES NOT BELIEVE THEY HAVE SCHIZOPHRENIA?

Schizophrenia can affect a person's thinking, feeling and behaviour. Sometimes the illness can even affect their ability to understand that they are ill. This is difficult for families who want their loved one to get help—and for the person with schizophrenia, who is being asked to seek help, but does not see the need.

Helping your relative to develop insight into their illness can take time. Be patient, and encourage your family member to talk about their feelings. If the person is resistant to talking about the illness, start with an area of their life that is affected by the illness, and ask about ways to help. Families who have experienced this situation say that it is best not to challenge their family member's thoughts, but rather to work on a mutually agreed issue. Many people do develop insight into their illness, though some may not.

If your loved one appears to be struggling with symptoms but is not currently receiving treatment, just letting the person know that help exists may be enough to get them to seek treatment. For some people, it may take longer to accept that they have an illness that must be managed over their lifespan. Some people may experience several episodes of the illness before they consistently accept help from doctors and therapists.

It can be very difficult to watch the person who is ill struggle without trying to convince them to "take your medication" or "talk to your doctor." Repeated attempts to convince and cajole can lead to heated arguments and power struggles. If you are very close to the person with schizophrenia, and yet you feel that they may not be open to your observation that something is wrong, it may be more effective to have another trusted person approach them.

If you have your family member's permission to share information with their health care team, or if you are their substitute decision maker, collaborate with the health care team and your family member to help to the person learn about the illness and about recovery.

> In my role as a peer support worker, I've learned that people are at different stages of their recovery. Everyone's journey is as unique as the person. What works for one person may not work for another. Listening to the person to discover what kind of support is meaningful to them can make a big difference in developing trust and a safe space for the person to grow. — Moshe

WHAT CAN I DO TO HELP MY RELATIVE BECOME LESS ISOLATED?

Some people with schizophrenia may become isolated because the illness takes away their motivation. For others it may be because they experience paranoia and fear that others are trying to harm them. Whatever the reason, seeing your relative become isolated can be upsetting and hard to understand. Talk with your relative about how their isolation makes you feel, and ask what you can do to help them enjoy the company of others.

Structure, routine and meaning can help to build motivation and reduce isolation. Think of interests that your relative enjoys, for example, listening to or making music; being around dogs, cats or other animals; or following sports. Build activities around these interests. Some people may benefit from participating in local programs, volunteering (for example, at a gallery or theatre) or providing peer support to others with schizophrenia.

Your relative's treatment team may be able to help. If you have the person's permission to share information with the treatment team, or if you are the person's substitute decision maker, ask the team to work with you and your relative to understand why he or she is isolated, and to generate ideas for spending more time in the community. If your family member experiences paranoia, the treatment team may be able to suggest ways to decrease the person's distress and triggers.

There should be a support group to help parents become better advocates. — Gilda

WHAT SHOULD I DO IF MY FAMILY MEMBER IS DEPRESSED AND TALKS OF SUICIDE?

Some people with schizophrenia feel depressed, unlovable and hopeless. Occasionally, they may be in serious danger of taking their own lives.

People usually show warning signs that they are thinking of suicide before they attempt or die by suicide. If you can recognize suicidal thinking and other warning signs, you will be better prepared to act quickly and competently in times of crisis. Some of these warning signs are listed below.

People who are feeling suicidal may:
· show a sudden change in mood or behaviour
· show a sense of hopelessness and helplessness

- express the wish to die or end their life
- increase substance use
- withdraw from people and activities that they previously enjoyed
- experience changes in sleeping patterns
- have a decreased appetite
- give away prized possessions or make preparations for their death (for example, creating a will).

These signs should be taken seriously. Don't be afraid to ask your relative about thoughts or plans for suicide. Talk with your relative about what they are feeling, and encourage them to discuss suicidal feelings with their doctor or mental health professional. If immediate help is required and is not available, take your relative to the emergency department of the hospital where treatment was previously provided, or to the nearest general or psychiatric hospital. In the event of an emergency, call 911.

HOW CAN I SUPPORT MY FAMILY MEMBER IF THERE IS A CRISIS?

Dealing with a crisis is always easier when you are prepared. Communication can be difficult for a person in crisis, so ask your family member at a time when they are stable what comforts and supports would be most helpful in a crisis. Develop a safety plan with your relative to address any potential concerns in advance; this can reduce the level of stress for everyone involved. If you have access to your relative's treatment team, collaborate with them on the safety plan.

In the event of a crisis, bring your family member to the hospital. If additional support is needed, mobile health crisis teams may be available in your community by calling 911 and asking for mental health support. Otherwise, 911 can provide support in bringing your family member to the nearest hospital.

The following tips may help to avoid or de-escalate a crisis:

· Don't challenge delusions.
· Create a calm environment where your family member feels safe.
· Reduce stimulation such as TV, radio, music, computer games or other distractions.
· Don't shout, and don't criticize or insult your relative.
· Suggest activities or distractions that your relative has identified as helpful (e.g., music, breathing exercises, drawing).
· Give your relative physical space.
· Speak slowly and clearly, and use simple sentences.
· Invite your family member to sit down and talk to you about what is bothering him or her.[2]

How to support your family member

Having family and friends to turn to can improve your relative's quality of life, prevent isolation and help them to engage in the recovery process. Here are some ways to provide support:

· **Communicate openly and often with your family member.** To ensure that communication takes place and is effective, pick a time that is convenient for all involved, when everyone is calm. Set clear expectations: when family members understand what is expected from each other, it helps to decrease stress and conflict. Make sure the point of view of the family member with schizophrenia is made clear, and that everyone has an opportunity to contribute.

· **Keep emotional intensity at a lower level and avoid intense criticism.** People with schizophrenia can be sensitive to intense

---

2 Adapted with permission from: Schizophrenia Society of Canada. (2012). *Learning about Schizophrenia: Rays of Hope. A Reference Manual for Families and Caregivers* (4th rev. ed.). Winnipeg, MB: Author.

emotions in interactions, particularly when these emotions are negative and are linked to criticism. While this is true of many people, it can cause considerable distress for those with schizophrenia.

· **Help your relative to have a positive outlook for the future.** Focus on your relative's strengths and goals, rather than the illness. Identify factors that can help to protect them from relapse. Examples of protective factors include:
  - strong family and community support
  - limiting use of drugs and alcohol
  - getting the appropriate amount of sleep
  - reducing stress
  - taking medication as prescribed.

Work with your family member to identify these protective factors early on and help to keep them in place. Encourage the person to make and reach goals for the future.

· **Make sure your family member feels loved, supported, respected and valued.** Like anyone, people with schizophrenia need to feel accepted for who they are. Be careful to not spend all your time with your family member discussing treatment and recovery. At the same time, be sure the person knows you are there to support the recovery process.

· **Attend appointments with the treatment team.** If you have your relative's permission to share information with the treatment team, or if you are a substitute decision maker, you can provide helpful information to the treatment team. This includes information about your relative's symptoms and how they developed, and about their life and interests before the illness began. You can also learn from the team about the nature of the illness and treatment options, and work with the team and your relative to collaborate on a recovery plan.

· **Help your relative to connect with resources.** If your relative needs treatment, case management or other supports, help them to connect to services in your community. See page 68 for contact information for referral services and mental health agencies. Family doctors can also help with identifying mental health services and with the referral process.

· **Challenge stigma.** Public education campaigns encouraging people to talk openly about mental health have helped to correct myths about schizophrenia. But there are still many people who do not have an educated understanding of the illness. The media still portray people with schizophrenia in misleading ways— often showing them as violent, when statistics show that people with schizophrenia are more likely to be the victims of violence. Try not to let stigma allow you and your relative to become with-drawn, because this can hamper the recovery process. Educate yourself, your family member and others about the illness. Challenge stigma when you encounter it. Each time you do, you help your relative, and you help others with the illness.

· **Promote your relative's self-care and a healthy, active lifestyle.** The negative symptoms of schizophrenia can affect a person's ability to maintain hygiene and other basic self-care needs. While basic hygiene may be your relative's most obvious need, promot-ing a holistic approach to health may be the best way to ensure self-care. Emotional, spiritual and physical health all play a role in self-care. One way to promote self-care is to encourage positive coping mechanisms such as exercise and the pursuit of creative outlets. If substance use is an issue, it can trigger symptoms and have a negative impact on self-care. Helping your relative get the support needed to cut down or quit using substances can improve their overall health, including their self-care. Keep in mind that the pace of progress for improving health may be gradual, and is different for every person.

· **Help to ensure your relative takes medication as prescribed.**
Keeping to a medication routine can be challenging for some
people with schizophrenia. Medications help to manage symptoms
and to prevent further acute episodes of the illness. Work with
your relative to create and participate in a plan for taking medications as prescribed. Help the person to note any possible side-
effects of the medication or symptoms that are not managed by the
medication. These should be reported to the prescribing physician.

How to support yourself

Supporting your relative during recovery can be stressful, and is a
process that takes time. You may also need support. As the saying
goes, "Put your own oxygen mask on first," so you are in a better
position to help your relative and other family members with their
"masks." This will enable you to continue to be an active participant
in your relative's recovery.

Consider the following ways of supporting yourself as you provide
care and support to your relative:

· **Attend a support group.** Feelings of fear, uncertainty, isolation,
loss or grief are common to families of people with schizophrenia. Being with others who understand and experience similar
thoughts and emotions can be reassuring and helpful.

· **Educate yourself about the illness.** Learn all you can about schizophrenia, especially in the early stages of treatment. It will help
you to support your relative, and also to get the support you
need. The better informed you are about your relative's illness,
the better prepared you will be to navigate the treatment system
and to promote the person's recovery. A better understanding of

the illness can also help you come to terms with what it means to have a family member with schizophrenia. Just as important, knowing more will make it easier for you to talk about the illness and to educate others about how they can help to support your relative, and you.

· **Recognize your stress and learn coping mechanisms.** Family members need to find a balance between supporting their recovering relative and finding time for themselves. This helps to prevent exhaustion and burnout.

· **See a counsellor.** Sitting down with a counsellor, with or without your family member, can provide needed support. Professional counselling lets you express thoughts and feelings that you may not feel comfortable sharing with others, and allows you to feel that you're being heard. Counselling can also help you to improve your coping and communication skills; deal with feelings of depression, fear, anxiety and grief; and improve your sense of well-being. Counselling services may be available through your employer, if they offer an employee access program (EAP), or through a community hospital, clinic or mental health organization. You may also seek a counsellor or psychotherapist in private practice, whose fee may or may not be covered by employee benefits.

· **Practise self-care.** Self-care is important for everyone, especially when you are going through a difficult or stressful time. Make a point of taking care of your emotional, physical, spiritual and social needs.

· **Create boundaries.** Setting boundaries is as important as providing unconditional support. As a caregiver, you need to communicate your own needs and allow time for yourself. Setting firm and consistent definitions of unacceptable behaviour is crucial for the well-being and safety of everyone in the family. Having clear boundaries can provide a structured, predictable and secure environment for your relative.

> *Don't try to take on everything. You don't have to be the be-all and end-all. You think you have to be, but it's okay to just step back.* — Gilda

Working with mental health professionals

When your relative has given consent to your involvement in their care, or you have been assigned as the person's substitute decision maker, consider the following hints for working with mental health professionals:[3]

· Write things down (e.g., names, phone numbers, dates of meetings, questions).
· Ask for meetings with the treatment team—contact the unit social worker or outpatient case manager. When possible, include your family member in these meetings.
· Approach the staff if there are any concerns. If you do not receive a satisfactory response, contact the unit manager or the client relations co-ordinator. Staff will provide this information.
· Offer your own observations on your relative's progress, including any side-effects they may be experiencing and any medical or social history that might be relevant to how they are coping.
· When you contact a treatment team member, leave your name, contact number and a brief message outlining relevant questions or concerns.

---

3 Adapted from: Baker, S. & Martens, L. (2010). *Promoting Recovery from First Episode Psychosis: A Guide for Families*. Toronto: CAMH. p. 30.

- Respect your relative's wishes (e.g., how often you contact their treatment team).
- Ask for specific information. If you don't understand what you are being told, don't be embarrassed. Ask for clarification.

7 Explaining schizophrenia to children

Explaining schizophrenia and other mental illnesses to children can feel awkward and difficult. Sometimes parents will not tell their children that a family member has schizophrenia because they do not know how to explain it or they think the children will not understand. In an effort to protect children, they sometimes continue with family routines as if nothing was wrong.

The strategies of saying nothing and continuing with routines are difficult to maintain, and over time will be confusing to children trying to understand their relative's problem. Because children are sensitive and intuitive they will notice when a member of the family has emotional, mental and physical changes. Parents should avoid being secretive about the relative's schizophrenia, as children will develop their own—often wrong—ideas about their relative's condition.

Young children, especially those of preschool or elementary school age, tend to see the world as revolving around them. As a consequence, they blame themselves for unusual and upsetting events or changes in the family, or for unusual changes in other people. For example, if a child disobeys a parent and gets into trouble, and soon afterward the parent shows signs of distress or strange behaviour, the child may assume he or she is the cause of the parent's illness.

To explain schizophrenia to children, it is important to give them only as much information as they are mature or old enough to understand. Toddlers and preschool children can understand simple, short sentences, without much technical information. School-aged children can process more information, but may be overwhelmed by details about medications and therapies. Teenagers can manage most information, and often need to talk about what they see and feel. They may have questions about the genetics of schizophrenia and worry about getting the illness themselves. They may also have concerns about the stigma of mental illness. Sharing information with them provides an opening for discussion.

There are three main areas that are helpful for parents to cover when speaking with children about schizophrenia:

- **The parent or family member behaves this way because he or she has an illness.** It is easiest for children to understand schizophrenia when it is explained to them as an illness. You may explain it like this: "Schizophrenia is an illness, like a cold, except that you don't catch it, and rather than giving you a runny nose, it affects how people see, hear and think about things. For example, people with schizophrenia may hear voices that no one else can hear, or have strange thoughts and beliefs that are not real. Schizophrenia takes a long time to get better. People with schizophrenia need help from a doctor or therapist."

- **Reassure the child that he or she did not make the parent or family member get this illness.** Children need to know that their actions did not cause their loved one to develop the illness.

- **Reassure the child that the adults in the family and other people, such as doctors, are trying to help the affected person.** It is the responsibility of adults to take care of the family member with schizophrenia. Children should not worry about taking care of anyone who is ill. Children need their parents and other trusted adults to protect them. They should be allowed to talk about what they see and feel with someone who knows how hard it is for a relative to struggle with the symptoms of schizophrenia. The changes that occur in a loved one because of schizophrenia are often scary to children. They miss the time spent with the person who is ill.

Participating in activities outside the home helps children, as it exposes them to healthy relationships. As the relative with schizophrenia recovers, and they gradually resume family activities, this will help to improve their relationship with the children in the family.

If the relative with schizophrenia is a parent, they and the other parent should talk with the children about explaining schizophrenia to people outside the family. The support of friends is important for everyone. However, because schizophrenia can be hard to explain, and some families worry about the stigma of mental illness, family members will have to decide how open they wish to be about their situation.

Many parents and other family members with schizophrenia are able to have normal, loving relationships with children. However, there may be times when they are less patient and more easily irritated than usual. They may find it hard to tolerate the boisterous activities and noisy play that are part of children's everyday routine. For them, the family may have to design and develop structured routines to ensure that the person with schizophrenia has quiet and restful time away from situations that might worsen symptoms of the illness. Times should be planned to allow for children to play outside the home or for the family member with schizophrenia to rest for part of the day in a quiet area of the home.

When the relative with schizophrenia is in recovery, it helps for the person to explain their behaviour to the children. They may need to plan some special times with the children to re-establish their relationship and reassure the children that they are now more available.

More information on talking to children about psychosis-related illnesses is available in the pamphlet *When a Parent Has Psychosis . . . What Kids Want to Know*, available from the Centre for Addiction and Mental Health at www.camh.ca/en/education/about/camh_publications/Documents/Flat_PDFs/WAP_Psychosis.pdf.

Reference

Leamy, M., Bird, V., Le Boutillier, C., Williams, J. & Slade, M. (2011). Conceptual framework for personal recovery in mental health: Systematic review and narrative synthesis. *British Journal of Psychiatry*, *199* (6), 445–452.

Resources

WEBSITES

AMI-Quebec Action on Mental Illness
amiquebec.org

Canadian Mental Health Association
www.cmha.ca

Centre for Addiction and Mental Health
www.camh.ca

The International Hearing Voices Network
www.intervoiceonline.org

Mental Health Commission of Canada
www.mentalhealthcommission.ca

Ontario Mental Health Helpline
www.mentalhealthhelpline.ca

Peerzone
www.peerzone.info

Portico: Canada's Mental Health and Addiction Network
www.porticonetwork.ca

Psychiatric Patient Advocate Office
www.sse.gov.on.ca/mohltc/ppao

Rethink Mental Illness
www.rethink.org

Schizophrenia Society of Canada
www.schizophrenia.ca

Wellness Recovery Action Plan (WRAP)
http://mentalhealthrecovery.com

World Fellowship for Schizophrenia and Allied Disorders (WFSAD)
http://world-schizophrenia.org/

BOOKS AND PAMPHLETS

Baker, S. & Martens, L. (2010). *Promoting Recovery from First Episode Psychosis: A Guide for Families.* Toronto: Centre for Addiction and Mental Health.

Centre for Addiction and Mental Health. (2013). *Understanding Psychiatric Medications: Information for Consumers, Families and Friends.* Available: www.camh.ca/en/education/about/camh_publications/Pages/print_friendly_pdfs.aspx

Fuller Torrey, E. (2013). *Surviving Schizophrenia: A Family Manual* (6th ed). New York: HarperCollins.

Mueser, K.T. & Gingerich, S. (2006). *The Complete Guide to Schizophrenia: Helping Your Loved One Get the Most Out of Life.* New York: Guilford Press.

Other guides in this series

To order these and other CAMH publications,
contact CAMH Publications:

Toll-free: 1 800 661-1111
Toronto: 416 595-6059
E-mail: publications@camh.ca
Online store: http://store.camh.ca

Lightning Source UK Ltd.
Milton Keynes UK
UKHW021812190922
409103UK00008B/935